Fantastic a̶ ̶ ̶ ̶ ̶ ̶ ̶C̶h̶a̶i̶r̶ ̶Y̶o̶g̶a̶ ̶f̶o̶r̶ Seniors: A Beginner's Guide

Hello, My Dear Friends!

As we journey through the golden years of our lives, it's important to find activities that not only keep our bodies moving but also bring joy and vitality into our daily routines. That's why I'm thrilled to introduce you to the wonderful world of chair yoga, a gentle yet effective form of exercise that's perfectly suited for us seniors. Whether you're looking to improve your flexibility, build strength, or simply find a moment of peace in your busy day, chair yoga offers a path to wellness that is both accessible and enjoyable.

Imagine sitting comfortably in your chair, surrounded by the familiar comforts of home, as you embark on a journey of movement and mindfulness. Chair yoga is designed with you in mind, offering a way to engage in physical activity without the worry of getting down on the floor or balancing on one foot. It's about adapting the timeless practices of yoga to meet you where you are, making it an ideal choice for anyone, regardless of age, mobility, or experience with exercise.

The beauty of chair yoga lies in its simplicity and the profound impact it can have on your health and well-being. From stretching your muscles to calming your mind, each pose and sequence is an invitation to explore your body's potential and nurture your spirit. And the best part? You can start right where you are, using nothing more than a chair and your own breath.

In this guide, "Fantastic and Fun Chair Yoga for Seniors: A Beginner's Guide," we'll walk hand-in-hand through the basics of chair yoga, sharing stories of transformation, debunking common myths, and offering step-by-step instructions to help you build a practice that fits your life. Whether you're looking to ease stiffness, improve balance, or simply enjoy a moment of relaxation, chair yoga opens the door to a world of possibilities.

So, let's embrace this adventure together, with open hearts and a spirit of curiosity. Chair yoga isn't just about physical fitness; it's a celebration of what our bodies can do and a testament to the joy that movement brings. I invite you to join me in discovering the accessible, enriching practice of chair yoga, a practice that promises to enhance your daily life in ways you might never have imagined.

Welcome, my friends, to the start of a beautiful journey. Let's explore the joys and benefits of chair yoga together, finding strength, flexibility, and peace in every pose. Here's to embarking on a path that enriches our golden years with health, happiness, and a sense of wonder at all the things we can achieve.

Let the adventure begin!

Success Stories

In the vibrant tapestry of life, every thread tells a story, especially as we weave through the golden years. Among these threads are the heartwarming tales of seniors who have embraced chair yoga, transforming their lives in ways they never imagined. Let's share a few of these inspiring stories, each a testament to the power of gentle movement and mindful breathing.

Margaret's Journey to Joy

At 72, Margaret felt the weight of her years in her bones. The garden she once tended with love had grown wild, a symbol of the activities she let go due to her arthritis. Then, Margaret discovered chair yoga. Initially skeptical, she was soon marveling at the newfound flexibility in her joints. "Chair yoga gave me back my garden," she says with a smile. "And not just the one outside.

It revived the garden in my heart, the joy of living. Now, I move through my day with ease, bending and stretching, tending to my flowers and my soul."

David's Balance Restored

David, a retired teacher, found his world shrinking after a fall that shook his confidence. The fear of another fall kept him confined, his once adventurous spirit caged. Chair yoga entered his life as a beacon of hope. "It's not just about the physical balance," David reflects, "but the mental balance, too. Learning to trust my body again, to find strength in stillness and movement, has opened new doors. I walk with assurance now, my spirit as steady as my stride."

Eleanor's Quiet Revolution

For Eleanor, 68, anxiety was a constant companion, whispering worries and dimming the light of her days. Chair yoga seemed an unlikely ally, yet it proved to be her fortress of calm. "Each pose, each breath, felt like a whisper telling me, 'It's going to be okay,'" Eleanor shares. "I found peace in the rhythm of my breathing, a quiet revolution against the noise of my anxieties. Chair yoga isn't just a practice for my body; it's therapy for my mind."

George's Second Wind

George, a veteran, carried the legacy of his service not only in his heart but in his body's aches and pains. The thought of exercise was daunting until chair yoga showed him a gentler way to salute his strength. "I've served my country, and now I'm learning to serve myself," George says, his voice a blend of pride and humility. "Chair yoga has been my second wind. My mornings start with gratitude and movement, honoring what my body can do. It's my daily act of service to myself, my personal victory."

Anna's Social Butterfly Emergence

Widowed and isolated, Anna, 75, longed for connection but didn't know where to start. Chair yoga became more than a physical activity; it was her bridge to others. "Joining a chair yoga group online, I found a community," Anna beams. "We share more than yoga; we share our lives. I've made friends who encourage me, laugh with me, and grow with me. Chair yoga brought me out of my cocoon, and I've emerged a social butterfly, fluttering with joy."

Each of these stories shines a light on the transformative power of chair yoga. Margaret, David, Eleanor, George, and Anna are but a few of the many seniors who have found in chair yoga a path to renewed strength, balance, peace, and connection. Their journeys remind us that it's never too late to start, to change, to grow. Through chair yoga, they've woven new threads of joy and vitality into the tapestry of their lives, inspiring us all to embrace each day with open hearts and the courage to transform.

The Benefits Explained

Embarking on the journey of chair yoga opens up a world of benefits tailored to meet the unique needs of us seniors. It's like finding a key to unlock potential we might not have known we had, gently nudging our bodies and minds towards better health and happiness. Let's dive into the simple yet profound ways chair yoga can enrich our lives, especially as we savor the golden years.

Flexibility: The Gentle Stretch

As we age, our muscles and joints may whisper (or sometimes shout) complaints a bit more loudly than they used to. Chair yoga steps in as a gentle friend, offering stretches that don't ask too much, yet give back in abundance. Imagine reaching up to the sky, feeling a stretch along your sides, or twisting gently from the comfort of your chair, loosening the stiffness that comes from sitting or less activity. These movements encourage our bodies to become more pliable, reducing the risk of injuries and making daily tasks easier and more enjoyable. Flexibility isn't just about touching our toes; it's about extending our reach towards a life lived with more ease.

Strength: Building from Within

Strength in our senior years isn't about lifting heavy weights; it's about empowering our bodies to lift us through life's daily challenges. Chair yoga introduces strength building in a way that's both doable and enjoyable. Each pose engages specific muscle groups, from our arms and shoulders to our core and legs, without any strain. Over time, these gentle exercises can significantly enhance our muscle tone and endurance, making us feel stronger and more capable. It's about giving us the strength to carry groceries, play with grandchildren, and enjoy hobbies without the shadow of weakness.

Balance: A Steady Confidence

Balance is a precious commodity that can wane as the years pass, but chair yoga offers a beautiful way to reclaim it. Through focused movements and poses, we learn to distribute our weight evenly, improving our posture and steadiness. This practice translates into fewer falls and a more confident stride, whether we're navigating the cobblestones of a cherished vacation spot or the steps of our own homes. Beyond the physical, chair yoga enhances our inner balance, instilling a sense of calm and assurance that steadies us in life's unpredictable moments.

Mental Health: The Peaceful Mind

Perhaps one of the most significant gifts chair yoga offers is the serenity it brings to our minds. The practice intertwines movement with breath, guiding us into a state of mindfulness that quiets the chatter of daily worries and stresses. This peaceful engagement has profound effects, from alleviating symptoms of anxiety and depression to enhancing sleep quality. Imagine ending a session of chair yoga feeling not just physically rejuvenated but mentally refreshed, carrying that tranquility into every corner of your day. It's about finding a sanctuary of peace within ourselves, a shelter we can always turn to.

Tailoring to Senior Needs

Chair yoga understands the melody of our senior years, composing movements that respect our rhythms and challenges. It offers modifications to accommodate health issues, ensuring that everyone can participate and benefit, regardless of physical limitations. This inclusivity is the heart of chair yoga, making it a practice that truly belongs to us seniors, one that celebrates our journey with every gentle stretch, strengthening pose, and balanced breath.

In embracing chair yoga, we don't just adopt a series of exercises; we welcome a companion that walks with us towards a horizon of well-being. It's a practice that weaves flexibility, strength, balance, and mental peace into the fabric of our daily lives, enhancing our golden years with the richness of health and joy.

Debunking Myths

As we meander through the golden years, it's not uncommon to encounter myths and misconceptions that might deter us from trying new activities, especially something as seemingly youthful as yoga. However, when it comes to chair yoga, many of these myths couldn't be further from the truth. Let's unravel some of these misconceptions together, illuminating the path for a journey that is indeed for everyone, no matter the age or stage in life.

Myth 1: Yoga is Only for the Young and Flexible

One of the most pervasive myths is the idea that yoga is reserved for the young, those who can twist themselves into pretzels with ease. This couldn't be more misleading. Chair yoga is specifically designed with us seniors in mind, celebrating our capabilities while gently nudging our limitations. It's not about performing complex poses but about engaging in a practice that enhances flexibility at any level. The beauty of chair yoga lies in its adaptability, making yoga accessible to all ages and flexibility levels. Remember, flexibility is not a prerequisite; it's a benefit that grows with practice.

Myth 2: You Need to Be Physically Fit to Do Yoga

Another common misconception is that one must already be in peak physical condition to participate in yoga. This notion overlooks the inclusive nature of chair yoga, which is crafted to build physical fitness, not demand it upfront. Chair yoga meets you where you are, transforming your chair into a supportive tool that helps improve strength, flexibility, and balance over time. Whether you're managing chronic conditions or simply haven't exercised in a while, chair yoga is a gentle gateway to enhancing your physical well-being, step by step.

Myth 3: Yoga Doesn't Offer Real Health Benefits

Some may dismiss yoga, and chair yoga by extension, as merely a relaxing pastime rather than a genuine health-enhancing activity. This myth fails to recognize the wealth of scientific research supporting yoga's benefits for both body and mind. From reducing blood pressure and improving heart health to easing anxiety and promoting better sleep, the health benefits of chair yoga are both real and profound. It's a holistic approach to wellness that nurtures not just the physical body but also the mental and emotional selves.

Myth 4: Yoga Requires Special Equipment and Clothing

The image of a yoga studio filled with expensive mats, blocks, and attire can be intimidating, suggesting that yoga necessitates a high investment in gear. Chair yoga, however, strips down these barriers, emphasizing simplicity and accessibility. All you really need is a sturdy chair and comfortable clothing that allows for movement. There's no need for specialized equipment or fancy yoga wear; chair yoga is about making the most of what you have, where you are.

Myth 5: It's Too Late to Start Yoga

Perhaps the most disheartening myth is the belief that there's an expiration date on starting a yoga practice. Let's clear the air once and for all: it is never too late to start chair yoga. This practice is a testament to the timeless truth that we are always capable of growth, learning, and transformation. Chair yoga is a celebration of what the body can do at any age, offering a practice that enhances quality of life, regardless of when you begin.

By debunking these myths, we uncover the truth that chair yoga is a welcoming, beneficial, and accessible practice for seniors. It's a gentle reminder that our golden years can be a time of discovery, growth, and renewal. So, let's cast aside these misconceptions and step confidently onto the path of chair yoga, embracing the journey with open hearts and minds. It's a journey that promises not just improved physical health but a deeper connection to the joy and vitality that dwell within us, waiting to be explored.

Creating Your Space

Creating a comfortable and safe space for your chair yoga practice at home is like setting the stage for a personal retreat, a sanctuary where you can explore movement, breath, and tranquility. This special spot doesn't need to be large or elaborate; with a few thoughtful touches, any corner of your home can become the perfect backdrop for your yoga journey. Here's how to create a nurturing environment that invites relaxation and focus, enhancing your chair yoga experience.

1. Choose a Quiet Corner

Look for a quiet area in your home where interruptions are minimal. This could be a corner of your living room, a spare bedroom, or even a peaceful spot on your enclosed porch. The key is finding a place where you can be undisturbed for the duration of your practice. A tranquil environment helps in cultivating a state of mindfulness and presence, allowing you to fully immerse yourself in the experience.

2. Ensure Ample Space

While chair yoga doesn't require a lot of room, you'll want to make sure there's enough space for you to move your arms freely, perhaps extend your legs, and rotate your body without bumping into furniture. A clear area around your chair ensures safety and ease of movement. You don't need a vast expanse; just ensure you can stretch out a bit without constraints.

3. Select a Supportive Chair

The centerpiece of your chair yoga space is, of course, the chair. Choose one that is sturdy and comfortable, with a firm seat that allows your feet to rest flat on the ground. Avoid chairs with wheels or those that are too soft and cushy, as they may not provide the stability you need. A good chair supports your posture and enhances your ability to engage in the poses confidently.

4. Gather Props You May Need

While chair yoga can be done with just a chair, you might find certain props helpful. Items like yoga blocks, a strap, or a cushion can be used to modify poses or support your body. Keeping these props within reach in your yoga space means you can easily incorporate them into your practice as needed, without having to interrupt your flow to search for them.

5. Create a Pleasant Atmosphere

Consider the ambiance of your yoga space. Natural light, a few plants, or a view of your garden can add a refreshing, calming element to your practice. If you enjoy, you might include a small speaker for soft music or the soothing sounds of nature. Some find that a favorite piece of art or a simple altar with items that inspire peace and happiness—like photos, candles, or stones—enhances the atmosphere, making the space feel personal and inviting.

6. Ensure Good Lighting

Good lighting is essential, not just for creating a pleasant environment but also for helping you see clearly as you follow along with yoga videos or read from a yoga guide. Natural light is wonderful, but if that's not available, ensure your space is well-lit with gentle, non-glaring lights.

7. Maintain Safety and Accessibility

Make sure your yoga area is easy to access, especially if mobility is a concern. Keep the floor clear of any rugs or cords that could pose a trip hazard, and have a clear path to your yoga spot. Safety is paramount, ensuring that your practice is both enjoyable and free from the risk of injury.

Creating your chair yoga space is an act of self-care, a way to honor your commitment to your well-being. This personal sanctuary becomes a sacred place where you can explore the benefits of chair yoga, cultivating strength, flexibility, balance, and peace. With your space set up, you're ready to embark on your chair yoga journey, embracing the practice as a cherished part of your daily routine.

Choosing Your Chair

Selecting the right chair for your chair yoga practice is akin to finding the perfect dance partner: it should support you flawlessly through every move, providing stability without overshadowing your grace. The chair becomes an extension of your body, offering a secure foundation from which you can explore various poses and sequences. Here's a guide to choosing a chair that will not only keep you safe but also enhance your yoga experience, making it comfortable and rewarding.

1. Look for Stability

The most crucial feature of your chair yoga companion is stability. You want a chair that feels as steady as the ground beneath you, one that won't wobble or tip as you shift your weight or try different poses. A chair with four solid legs is typically more stable than those with wheels or a swivel base. Test the chair by sitting in it and gently moving side to side and forward and back. If it feels secure and doesn't slide or tip easily, it's a good candidate.

2. Consider the Height

The ideal chair height is one where you can sit with your feet flat on the floor and your knees at a comfortable 90-degree angle. This position promotes good posture and alignment, which are essential in yoga practice. If you're on the taller or shorter side, take some time to find a chair that matches your proportions. Remember, a chair that's too high can strain your thighs and lower back, while one that's too low can make it harder to rise or perform certain movements.

3. Check the Seat Depth and Width

A chair that's too deep can make it difficult to sit properly with your back against the chair's backrest, while one that's too narrow may feel constricting or uncomfortable. Look for a chair with a seat that allows you to sit comfortably with your back supported and a little space between the edge of the seat and the back of your knees. This ensures proper circulation and makes it easier to maintain good posture during your practice.

4. Avoid Armrests if Possible

While armrests can be comfortable for sitting, they might limit your range of motion during chair yoga. They can interfere with side stretches, twists, or arm movements. If possible, choose a chair without armrests for the greatest flexibility in your practice. However, if armrests are necessary for your comfort or stability when sitting and standing, ensure they don't hinder your ability to perform most of the poses you wish to incorporate into your practice.

5. Seek Comfort, But Not Too Much

Your chair should be comfortable enough to sit in for the duration of your yoga session but not so plush that it compromises your stability. A chair with a firm, flat seat is ideal. It provides the support needed for proper alignment and makes it easier to engage your core muscles. A little padding can add comfort, but avoid chairs that are too soft or that cause you to sink down and slouch.

6. Material Matters

Consider the material of your chair, especially if you'll be practicing in shorts or sleeveless tops. Metal or plastic chairs can feel cold or slippery, while upholstered chairs offer more warmth and grip but can be harder to clean. Look for a material that feels pleasant against your skin and offers a balance of comfort and practicality.

7. Personalize Your Choice

Finally, remember that the best chair for you is one that meets your unique needs and preferences. It might take a bit of searching to find the perfect match, but the effort is well worth it. Your chair is more than just a piece of furniture; it's a tool that supports your journey towards greater health and well-being.

By choosing the right chair for your chair yoga practice, you set the stage for a safe, enjoyable, and effective experience. This chair becomes your steady ally, a trusted support that allows you to explore the depths of your practice with confidence and grace.

What You Need

Embarking on your chair yoga journey is an exciting adventure, one that requires very little in terms of equipment. However, a few optional items can enhance your practice, offering support, increasing accessibility, and helping you to deepen certain poses. Here's a straightforward list of these items and how they can be integrated into your chair yoga routine for a more fulfilling experience.

1. Yoga Blocks

Yoga blocks can be incredibly versatile, acting as extensions of your arms or providing support for various poses. For instance, if you're doing a side stretch and can't quite reach the floor comfortably, placing a block under your hand can bring the ground up to you. Blocks are great for maintaining alignment and ensuring comfort, especially in poses that require a little extra reach or stability.

2. Yoga Strap

A yoga strap (or a belt or a scarf if you're improvising) can help you achieve poses that involve stretching the legs or arms. For example, if you're working on a leg stretch and can't comfortably hold your foot with your hand, wrapping a strap around your foot and holding the ends can make the pose accessible. Straps are excellent for gently enhancing flexibility over time, allowing you to maintain proper form without straining.

3. Yoga Mat

While not essential for chair yoga, a yoga mat can be useful if you're incorporating standing poses that require you to step off the chair or if you're practicing on a slippery surface. A mat provides traction under your feet, ensuring safety and stability during your practice.

4. Cushions or Pillows

Cushions or pillows can make your chair yoga practice more comfortable. For instance, placing a cushion on the seat of your chair can offer extra padding for seated poses. Similarly, a small pillow behind your back can provide additional support during backbends or twists, ensuring that you maintain good posture without straining.

5. Blanket

A folded blanket can serve multiple purposes in chair yoga. It can be used to adjust the height of your seat by sitting on it, to support your feet if they don't quite reach the floor, or to keep you warm during relaxation poses. Blankets offer a simple way to customize your practice to your body's needs, ensuring comfort and proper alignment.

6. Lightweight Dumbbells or Water Bottles

For those looking to add a bit of strength training to their chair yoga routine, lightweight dumbbells or even a pair of filled water bottles can be used. They can be incorporated into arm raises or twists to build muscle tone. This is optional and should be approached with caution, focusing on maintaining good form and avoiding strain.

7. Relaxation Aids

Items like lavender eye pillows, essential oil diffusers, or soft music can enhance the relaxation aspect of your chair yoga practice. These aids can help create a soothing environment, making the transition into relaxation or meditation poses more immersive.

Remember, these items are entirely optional. Chair yoga can be practiced effectively with just a chair and your willingness to explore movement and breath. However, incorporating one or more of these items can tailor the experience to your personal needs, preferences, and goals, making your practice even more enjoyable and beneficial.

Seated Mountain Pose

This pose is perfect for beginners and offers a great way to start your practice, focusing on posture, breath, and the serene engagement of your body and mind.

1. Start by Sitting Properly: Sit in the middle of your chair with your feet flat on the floor, hip-distance apart. Ensure your chair is stable and without arms for unrestricted movement. Your knees should be aligned directly over your ankles, creating a straight line from your shoulders to your hips.

2. Align Your Spine: Place your hands on your thighs, palms down. Engage your abdominal muscles slightly to support your spine. Imagine a string attached to the top of your head, gently pulling you upwards, elongating your spine and lifting your chest.

3. Relax Your Shoulders: Roll your shoulders up towards your ears, then gently back and down. This helps release

tension in your neck and shoulders, fostering an open, relaxed posture.

4. Focus on Your Breath: Close your eyes or soften your gaze, directing your attention inward. Take a few deep, slow breaths, inhaling through your nose and exhaling through your mouth. With each breath, feel yourself becoming more centered and grounded.

5. Engage Your Entire Body: Even though you are seated, engage your legs as if you were standing on the ground. Press your feet firmly into the floor, activating your leg muscles. Feel the stability and strength of your body in this pose.

6. Hold and Breathe: Maintain the Seated Mountain Pose for several breaths, aiming for deep, even breaths. With each inhale, imagine growing taller; with each exhale, feel your body grounding further into your chair.

7. Release the Pose: When you're ready to release the pose, relax your hands and take a moment to notice any changes in your body or mind. The Seated Mountain Pose

is an excellent way to cultivate a sense of calm and presence, preparing you for further poses or the rest of your day.

8. This pose is a cornerstone of chair yoga, emphasizing the importance of posture and breathing in creating a foundation for your practice. Through regular engagement, you'll find yourself more attuned to your body's needs and capabilities, ready to explore more poses with confidence and ease.

Seated Cat-Cow Stretch

Let's explore the Seated Cat-Cow Stretch, a dynamic duo of poses that brings flexibility to the spine, promotes deep breathing, and encourages gentle movement between two contrasting postures.

1. Begin in a Seated Position: Sit towards the front of your chair, ensuring it is stable and without arms for ease of movement. Place your feet flat on the floor, hip-width

apart. Rest your hands on your knees or the tops of your thighs.

2. Move into Cow Pose: Inhale deeply, arch your back, and tilt your pelvis forward to accentuate the curve of your lower back. Lift your chin slightly, opening your chest, and gently push your shoulders back. This position encourages a gentle stretch across your chest and throat and a subtle engagement of your back muscles.

3. Transition to Cat Pose: On an exhale, round your spine, tuck your chin to your chest, and gently lean back, pushing your spine towards the chair back. Pull your belly button towards your spine, engaging your abdominal muscles. This pose stretches the muscles of your back and neck, providing a counterbalance to the Cow stretch.

4. Flow Between Poses: Alternate between Cow Pose on your inhales and Cat Pose on your exhales, moving at the pace of your own breath. This flowing movement helps to lubricate and stretch the spine while encouraging deep, rhythmic breathing.

5. Focus on the Spine: As you move between these poses, concentrate on the sensations in your spine. Notice the gentle stretching and releasing of the muscles along your back. Allow the movement to be smooth and fluid, without any sharp movements or strain.

6. Continue the Sequence: Repeat the Cat-Cow Stretch several times, following the rhythm of your breath. This repetition enhances spinal flexibility and brings a sense of relaxation to the body and mind.

7. Conclude with Stillness: After completing the sequence, return to a neutral, seated position. Take a moment to breathe deeply and observe any changes in your body or mind. The Seated Cat-Cow Stretch is not only about physical movement but also about connecting with your breath and cultivating a mindful awareness of the present moment.

This sequence is a gentle yet effective way to warm up the body, making it a perfect starting point for a chair yoga practice or a standalone routine to relieve tension and enhance spinal health. Through regular practice, you'll notice increased mobility in your spine and a deeper connection between your movements and your breath.

Seated Forward Bend

Moving forward in our exploration of basic chair yoga poses, let's focus on the Seated Forward Bend. This pose is a fantastic way to stretch the spine and shoulders, encourage relaxation, and promote introspection.

1. Starting Position: Sit at the edge of a sturdy, armless chair with your feet firmly planted on the ground, hip-width apart. Sit up tall, aligning your head, neck, and spine, and place your hands on your thighs or knees.

2. Initiate the Bend: Inhale deeply, lengthening your spine as if reaching up through the crown of your head. As you exhale, slowly hinge at your hips, not your waist, to bend forward. This mindful movement ensures that the bend originates from your hip joints, providing a deeper stretch and protecting your back.

3. Deepen the Pose: Continue to fold forward, allowing your hands to slide down your legs towards your feet. Keep your neck in a neutral position, in line with your spine, and let your head and arms hang freely towards the floor. The goal is not to reach your toes but to find a comfortable stretch in your back and legs.

4. Hold and Breathe: Once you've reached a comfortable depth, hold the position for several breaths. With each inhale, imagine lengthening your spine; with each exhale, gently deepen into the bend. This breathing pattern helps to relax the body further into the pose, enhancing the stretch and calming the mind.

5. Engage Your Core: Throughout the pose, maintain a slight engagement of your abdominal muscles. This support for your lower back ensures the stretch is beneficial and safe, preventing any strain.

6. Return to Seated Position: To come out of the pose, slowly roll your spine up, one vertebra at a time, on an inhale. Your head should come up last, returning you to a seated position with a straight spine. Take a moment to notice any sensations in your body, embracing the feeling of openness and relaxation.

7. Modifications: If bending forward is challenging, you can place a cushion or yoga block on your lap to rest your hands or elbows on, reducing the intensity of the stretch. This modification allows you to enjoy the benefits of the pose without discomfort.

The Seated Forward Bend is a beautiful expression of inward focus and physical stretch. It offers a moment of pause in your practice to reflect and breathe, gently stretching the back and promoting a state of calm. Regular practice of this pose can improve flexibility, reduce stress, and enhance overall well-being, making it a cherished part of any chair yoga routine.

Seated Spinal Twist

Continuing our exploration of foundational chair yoga poses, let's delve into the Seated Spinal Twist. This pose is excellent for increasing spinal mobility, stretching the shoulders, and stimulating digestion.

1. Position Your Chair: Begin by sitting sideways on your chair, ensuring it's stable and without arms for ease of movement. If your chair has a back, position it to the side of your body that you'll be twisting towards.

2. Set Your Foundation: Plant your feet firmly on the ground, hip-width apart. If you're twisting to the right, your right leg should be bent with the foot flat on the ground, and your left leg extended slightly

forward to keep the hips square and stable.

3. Initiate the Twist: Place your right hand on the back of the chair and your left hand on your right knee. Inhale deeply to lengthen your spine, imagining a straight line reaching up through the crown of your head.

4. Deepen the Twist: As you exhale, gently twist your torso to the right, using your hands as leverage to deepen the twist without forcing it. Keep your spine tall and your shoulders relaxed. Your gaze can follow the direction of the twist, encouraging a gentle neck stretch.

5. Hold and Breathe: Maintain the twist for several deep breaths, focusing on lengthening the spine with each inhale and deepening the twist with each exhale.

This breathing pattern helps to maximize the stretch and the benefits of the pose.

6. Release and Repeat: To come out of the twist, slowly return your torso to the front on an inhale, releasing your hands back to your lap. Pause for a moment to notice any sensations, then switch the direction of your chair and repeat the twist on the opposite side to maintain balance in your body.

7. Modifications and Cautions: If you have any back or spine issues, it's important to approach this pose with caution and perhaps consult with a healthcare provider or a yoga instructor specialized in chair yoga for modifications that can suit your individual needs.

The Seated Spinal Twist is a versatile pose that can be easily incorporated into any chair yoga practice. It offers numerous benefits, including improving spinal flexibility, aiding in digestion, and relieving tension in the back and shoulders. Regular practice can contribute to a greater sense of overall well-being, highlighting the pose's importance in a balanced chair yoga routine.

Seated Leg Extension

Our journey through foundational chair yoga poses brings us to the Seated Leg Extension, a simple yet effective stretch that targets the hamstrings and encourages flexibility in the legs.

1. Start in a Seated Position: Sit on the edge of a stable, armless chair with your feet flat on the ground. Ensure your back is straight, shoulders relaxed, and your core slightly engaged for support.

2. Prepare for the Extension: Begin with both feet planted on the ground. Sit up tall, engaging your core to support your spine.

3. Extend One Leg: Gently extend one leg forward, keeping the heel on the ground and toes pointing upwards. The other foot should remain flat on the floor, providing stability and balance.

4. Position Your Hands: Place your hands on the thigh of the bent leg, using them for support but not leaning forward. Your back should remain straight, aligning your spine over your hips.

5. Focus on the Stretch: As you sit tall, gently press the heel of your extended leg into the ground, feeling a stretch along the back of your leg. Keep your toes flexed towards you to intensify the stretch in the hamstring and calf muscles.

6. Hold and Breathe: Maintain this position for several deep breaths, focusing on relaxing into the stretch without straining. With each exhale, see if you can

deepen the stretch slightly, always listening to your body's limits.

7. Release and Repeat: To release the pose, slowly bend your extended leg, bringing your foot back to the floor. Take a moment to notice any differences between your legs before switching sides and repeating the stretch with the other leg extended.

8. Modifications: If you find it challenging to keep your leg straight, it's perfectly fine to have a slight bend in the knee. The key is to feel a gentle stretch in the back of the leg, not to force the leg into straightness.

The Seated Leg Extension is a wonderfully accessible pose that offers multiple benefits, including improved leg flexibility, enhanced circulation, and relief from stiffness in the hamstrings and calves. Regular practice can lead to greater mobility and comfort in daily activities, making it a valuable addition to any chair yoga practice.

Seated Eagle Arms

Continuing our exploration of basic chair yoga poses for beginners, let's delve into the Seated Eagle Arms, a pose that focuses on stretching the shoulders, upper back, and arms. This pose is particularly beneficial for relieving tension in the upper body, a common area of discomfort for many. It can be easily adapted to suit any level of flexibility, making it a versatile addition to your chair yoga practice.

1. Begin in a Comfortable Seat: Sit upright in your chair with your feet flat on the ground, hip-width apart. Ensure your back is straight but not rigid, and your shoulders are relaxed down away from your ears.

2. Cross Your Arms: Extend your arms straight in front of you at shoulder height. Cross your right arm over your left, bending both elbows. The right elbow will nestle into the crook of the left. If possible, bring your palms to touch, or as close together as comfortable. If this is not accessible, simply press the backs of your hands together or hold onto your shoulders for a bear hug position.

3. Lift and Stretch: With your arms crossed and bent, lift your elbows to the height of your shoulders while gently pressing your hands forward away from your face. This action creates a broadening and stretching sensation across your upper back and shoulders.

4. Hold and Breathe: Maintain this pose for several deep breaths. Focus on relaxing your shoulders away from your ears even as you stretch. With each exhale, see if you

can deepen the stretch slightly, always respecting your body's limits and never forcing the pose.

5. Release and Repeat on the Other Side: To release the pose, gently unwind your arms and extend them out to the sides on an inhale. On an exhale, cross your left arm over your right and repeat the pose with the arms switched to balance the stretch on both sides of your body.

6. Modifications: If crossing your arms fully is challenging, focus on the bear hug variation by simply wrapping your arms around your shoulders. This modification still provides a beneficial stretch to the shoulders and upper back without the need for full arm entanglement.

The Seated Eagle Arms pose is an excellent way to address the stiffness and tension that can accumulate in the upper body, especially for those who spend a lot of time sitting or engaging in repetitive tasks. By incorporating this pose into your chair yoga routine, you can enjoy increased mobility in your shoulders, improved posture, and a significant reduction in upper body stress. Regular practice of the Seated Eagle Arms can enhance your overall well-being and contribute to a more balanced and comfortable physical state.

Seated Side Stretch

Introducing the Seated Side Stretch, an essential pose for beginners in chair yoga that focuses on elongating the side body, enhancing flexibility, and promoting better breathing.

1. Start in a Seated Position: Begin by sitting upright in a chair without arms, ensuring your feet are flat on the ground and hip-width apart. Engage your core slightly to support your spine.

2. Initiate the Stretch: Place your left hand on the left side of the chair for stability. Inhale and extend your right arm straight up beside your ear, keeping your shoulder relaxed away from your ear.

3. Lean to the Side: As you exhale, gently lean your torso to the left, keeping your right arm extended overhead. The movement should come from your waist, creating a gentle curve on your right side. Ensure both hips remain firmly planted on the chair to maintain balance and maximize the stretch.

4. Deepen the Stretch: Reach through your right fingertips to intensify the stretch along your right side. Keep your chest and shoulders open, avoiding the tendency to lean forward or back. Your gaze can follow the direction of your stretch or remain forward, depending on your comfort.

5. Hold and Breathe: Stay in this position for a few deep breaths, focusing on lengthening the side of your body with each inhale and deepening the stretch with each exhale. The breath will help you find more space in the stretch and ease any tension.

6. Return to Center and Repeat: To come out of the stretch, inhale and lift your torso back to an upright position, lowering your right arm. Pause for a moment to notice the sensations in your body before switching sides. Repeat the stretch on the opposite side to ensure balance in your body.

The Seated Side Stretch is a beautifully accessible pose for individuals at any level of fitness or flexibility. It's particularly beneficial for opening up the ribcage, which can improve breathing capacity and aid in releasing tension in the back and shoulders. Regular practice can lead to increased mobility in the spine and a greater sense of overall well-being. The tranquil setting and focused posture depicted in the illustration serve as a reminder of the peaceful and rejuvenating nature of chair yoga, making it an ideal practice for enhancing quality of life.

Seated Ankle-to-Knee Pose

Introducing the Seated Ankle-to-Knee Pose, a wonderful stretch for beginners in chair yoga that targets the hips, promoting flexibility and reducing tightness.

1. Start in a Seated Position: Sit towards the edge of a chair without arms, ensuring your back is straight and your feet are flat on the ground. This initial posture helps in maintaining balance and alignment throughout the pose.

2. Position Your Legs: Gently lift your left foot and place your left ankle on your

right knee, creating a figure-four shape with your legs. Keep your right foot grounded to provide stability.

3. Adjust Your Pose: Rest your hands on your left shin or thigh, depending on what feels most comfortable, while keeping your spine elongated. This not only aids in maintaining balance but also helps deepen the stretch without straining.

4. Deepen the Stretch: To intensify the stretch in your hip and gluteal area, you can gently lean forward from your hips, keeping your back straight. Remember, the goal is to feel a gentle opening in the hip, not to push to the point of discomfort.

5. Hold and Breathe: Maintain this pose for several deep breaths, focusing on relaxing your hip muscles with each exhale. The

breath plays a crucial role in releasing tension and facilitating a deeper stretch.

6. Release and Switch Sides: To come out of the pose, carefully lift your left leg off your right knee and place your foot back on the ground. Pause for a moment to observe any sensations before repeating the stretch on the opposite side, placing your right ankle on your left knee.

The Seated Ankle-to-Knee Pose is an accessible and effective way to address hip tightness, a common issue among seniors. The cozy and inviting atmosphere depicted in the illustration, complete with ambient lighting and a cup of tea, mirrors the nurturing and gentle approach of chair yoga to improving flexibility and well-being. By incorporating this pose into your routine, you can enjoy the benefits of a more open and flexible lower body, contributing to improved mobility and comfort in daily activities.

Seated Chest Opener

For beginners embracing the journey of chair yoga, the Seated Chest Opener is an essential pose that promotes better posture, relieves tension in the upper body, and encourages deep breathing. This gentle exercise is perfect for counteracting the common issue of rounded shoulders, often a result of prolonged sitting or computer use. Let's walk through the steps to achieve this beneficial pose.

1. Begin in a Seated Position: Choose a sturdy, armless chair and sit with your feet flat on the ground, hip-width apart. Ensure your back is straight, aligning your spine over your hips. This posture forms the foundation of your chest opener.

2. Interlace Your Fingers: Extend your arms behind you and gently interlace your fingers. If directly interlacing them is challenging, you may grasp a small towel

or yoga strap between your hands to reduce the stretch intensity.

3. Open Your Chest: With your fingers interlaced, straighten your arms to the best of your ability. This action naturally encourages your shoulders to roll back and down, and your chest to lift and open. Be mindful to keep your chin parallel to the floor, maintaining a neutral neck position.

4. Deepen the Stretch: Gently squeeze your shoulder blades together, enhancing the opening across your chest. Ensure this movement is gentle and does not cause discomfort. The aim is to feel a comfortable stretch without straining.

5. Hold and Breathe: Maintain this position for several deep breaths. Focus on inhaling deeply to expand your chest further, and exhaling slowly to settle into

the stretch. Each breath helps to deepen the chest opening and release tension in the shoulders and neck.

6. Release with Care: To exit the pose, gently release your hands and bring your arms back to your sides. Take a moment to roll your shoulders softly, noticing any sensations of openness or relief in your upper body.

The Seated Chest Opener is an accessible and highly effective pose for enhancing upper body mobility and promoting a sense of openness and relaxation. It's an excellent practice for beginning or ending your chair yoga routine, offering benefits that extend beyond the mat, improving posture and comfort in daily activities.

Seated Forward Fold

Introducing the Seated Forward Fold, a fundamental pose in chair yoga suitable for beginners, focusing on stretching the spine, shoulders, and hamstrings. This pose offers a gentle way to release tension in the back and legs while promoting relaxation and stress relief. Here's how you can incorporate the Seated Forward Fold into your practice.

1. Start in a Seated Position: Sit at the edge of a sturdy, armless chair with your feet planted firmly on the ground, hip-width apart. Ensure your back is straight and your hands rest on your thighs.

2. Initiate the Fold: Inhale deeply and lengthen your spine, feeling as if a string is pulling you up from the crown of your head. As you exhale, hinge at your hips (not your waist) to fold forward slowly. This hinging motion is crucial for

protecting your back and deepening the stretch appropriately.

3. Deepen the Pose: Continue to fold forward, allowing your hands to slide down your legs towards your ankles or feet. Go only as far as comfortable without straining. Your goal is to feel a stretch in your back and hamstrings, not to reach your toes necessarily.

4. Relax Your Upper Body: Allow your head to hang loosely, releasing tension in your neck and shoulders. This relaxation is key to the pose, as it encourages a full spine stretch and provides a moment of rest and introspection.

5. Hold and Breathe: Stay in the forward fold for several deep breaths. With each inhale, imagine lengthening your spine; with each exhale, allow yourself to fold a

bit deeper, always within your comfort range.

6. Gently Return to Seated: To come out of the pose, slowly roll your spine up, vertebra by vertebra, on an inhale. Your head should come up last. Take a moment to sit upright and notice the sensations in your body.

The Seated Forward Fold is a versatile pose that can be easily modified to suit different flexibility levels. If reaching for your feet is challenging, consider holding onto your shins or simply letting your hands rest on the ground beside your chair. This pose is a wonderful addition to any chair yoga session, offering benefits like improved digestion, reduced anxiety, and increased flexibility in the back and legs. Regular practice can contribute to a greater sense of calm and physical well-being.

Seated Warrior II

Embarking on the journey of chair yoga, we discover the Seated Warrior II, a pose adapted from traditional standing yoga poses to suit beginners and those who prefer or require seated exercises. This pose emphasizes strengthening, stretching, and improving concentration. Seated Warrior II in a chair offers the benefits of its standing counterpart, focusing on the legs, arms, and core, while being accessible to individuals at all levels of mobility.

1. Start in a Seated Position: Sit in the middle of a sturdy, armless chair. If possible, choose a position where your back is not leaning against the chair back, promoting an active engagement of your core throughout the pose.

2. Position Your Legs: Extend your right leg out to the side, keeping your foot flat on the ground and your leg straight. Pivot

your left foot slightly, so it's still on the ground but angled comfortably, allowing your left knee to remain bent. This creates a foundation that mimics the stance of the traditional Warrior II pose but adapted for seated practice.

3. Align Your Arms: Extend your arms out to the sides at shoulder height, palms facing down. Your right arm should be reaching forward, parallel to your right leg, and your left arm extending back, creating a line of energy that runs through both fingertips.

4. Focus Your Gaze: Turn your head to look past your right fingertips, adopting the characteristic gaze (or "drishti") of the Warrior pose. This not only helps in maintaining balance but also enhances focus and determination.

5. Engage Your Core: While your legs and arms are actively engaged in the pose, remember to draw your abdominal muscles in towards your spine, supporting your upper body and maintaining a strong, upright posture.

6. Hold and Breathe: Maintain the Seated Warrior II pose for several deep breaths, feeling the stretch in your legs and arms, and the strength in your core. With each exhale, imagine sinking a little deeper into the pose, increasing the engagement of your muscles.

7. Release and Repeat: To release the pose, gently lower your arms and bring your right leg back to the starting position. Pause for a moment to notice the sensations in your body before switching sides, extending your left leg out and repeating the pose to ensure balance in your practice.

Seated Warrior II is a powerful pose that builds strength and stability while offering a moment of focused presence. It's a testament to the adaptability of yoga, proving that with modifications, the essence and benefits of traditional poses can be accessible to everyone, regardless of their physical condition. Incorporating Seated Warrior II into your chair yoga routine can enhance your physical strength, improve your flexibility, and foster a sense of inner warrior spirit.

Breathing Basics

Breathing is the essence of yoga and a powerful tool for enhancing relaxation and focus. In chair yoga, just as in traditional yoga, breathing exercises, or pranayama, play a crucial role in connecting the body and mind, helping to ease tension and cultivate a sense of peace. Here, we'll explore some simple breathing exercises designed for beginners, which can be incorporated into your chair yoga practice or used any time you need a moment of calm.

1. Diaphragmatic Breathing (Belly Breathing)

- How to Do It: Sit comfortably in your chair with your feet flat on the ground. Place one hand on your abdomen and the other on your chest. Inhale deeply through your nose, aiming to direct the breath down toward your stomach, feeling your hand rise. The hand on your chest should move very little. Exhale slowly through your mouth or nose, feeling your hand on your abdomen lower.

- Benefits: This type of breathing activates the parasympathetic nervous system, promoting relaxation and stress reduction. It's particularly effective for calming the mind and preparing for meditation.

2. Equal Breathing

- How to Do It: Sit up straight in your chair. Close your eyes to help focus inward. Inhale through your nose for a count of four, then exhale through your nose for a count of four. As you become comfortable, you can gradually increase the length of each inhale and exhale, ensuring they remain equal in duration.

- Benefits: This breathing technique is excellent for reducing anxiety, improving focus, and calming the mind. It's a simple yet powerful practice for creating balance in the body's energy systems.

3. Alternate Nostril Breathing

- How to Do It: Start by sitting comfortably with your back straight. Rest your left hand on your lap. Use your right hand to close off your right nostril with your thumb. Inhale slowly through your left nostril, then close it with your fingers. Open your right nostril and exhale slowly. Inhale through the right nostril, close it, and exhale through the left. This completes one cycle.

- Benefits: Alternate nostril breathing is known for its ability to balance the left and right hemispheres of the brain, enhance concentration, and reduce stress. It's a gentle way to refresh the mind and body.

4. The Humming Bee Breath

- How to Do It: Close your eyes and relax your face. You can place your fingers gently over your ears or simply rest your hands on your lap. Inhale deeply through your nose, then, as you exhale, make a gentle humming sound like a bee, feeling the vibration in your head.

- Benefits: This breathing exercise is particularly effective for soothing the nervous system, reducing stress and anxiety, and improving focus. The vibration of the hum can also help to quiet the mind.

Incorporating these simple breathing exercises into your daily routine can significantly enhance your relaxation, focus, and overall well-being. Whether as part of your chair yoga practice or as standalone techniques, they offer a readily accessible way to find calm and balance in the midst of a busy life. Remember, the key to pranayama is patience and consistency; with regular practice, you'll likely notice a profound impact on your mental and physical health.

Seasonal Sessions

Incorporating the essence of the seasons into your chair yoga practice can bring a refreshing and thematic touch to your routine, aligning your movements and breath with the natural world. Each season offers unique themes and inspirations that can enhance your practice, making it more engaging and meaningful. Here are some fun ideas for seasonal sessions to enrich your chair yoga experience.

Spring Renewal

Celebrate the season of new beginnings with poses and breathwork that emphasize renewal and growth. Focus on gentle stretching and opening poses that mimic the blossoming of flowers and the stretching of trees towards the light. Incorporate breathing exercises that emphasize clearing and rejuvenation, like deep, cleansing breaths. You might also introduce greenery into your practice space or practice near a window to connect with the budding life outside.

Summer Sunshine

Embrace the warmth and energy of summer with a practice that builds heat and fosters joy. Include poses that open the heart and stretch the front of the body, inviting in the sun's energy. Sun Salutations can be adapted to chair yoga, offering a dynamic sequence that warms the body. Breathing exercises can focus on energizing breaths, such as Kapalabhati (Skull Shining Breath). Consider practicing in a well-lit room or outdoors if possible, to physically soak in the sunshine.

Autumn Leaves

Autumn invites reflection and letting go, similar to the falling leaves. Incorporate twists and forward folds that symbolize releasing what no longer serves you. This season is perfect for practicing grounding poses that enhance stability and calmness, preparing the body and mind for the transition towards winter. For breathwork, focus on balancing techniques, like Nadi Shodhana (Alternate Nostril Breathing), to harmonize the body's energy as the season changes.

Winter Stillness

Winter, with its quiet and introspective energy, calls for a practice focused on stillness and inner warmth. Emphasize gentle, restorative poses that promote relaxation and warmth, such as seated cat-cow for spinal flexibility and seated forward bends for calmness. Use breathwork to build inner heat, like Ujjayi (Ocean Breath), and incorporate meditation or guided imagery focused on cozy, peaceful winter scenes to foster a sense of warmth and serenity.

Seasonal Themes and Decor

To fully embrace each season, consider integrating seasonal themes and decor into your practice space. This might include flowers in spring, bright colors in summer, leaves and earth tones in autumn, and soft, warm fabrics in winter. Seasonal essential oils or scents can also enhance the atmosphere, like floral scents for spring or cinnamon for winter.

By aligning your chair yoga practice with the cycles of nature, you not only add a rich layer of meaning to your routine but also deepen your connection to the natural world. Each season offers a unique opportunity to reflect, grow, and find balance, both on and off the chair.

Travel from Your Chair

"Travel from Your Chair" is a delightful concept in chair yoga that invites imagination and movement to merge, offering a unique way to explore the world and its diverse landscapes without leaving your home. By incorporating imaginative sequences into your chair yoga practice, you can embark on journeys that not only enhance your physical well-being but also enrich your mental and emotional landscapes. Here are some creative ideas to take you on global adventures and nature excursions from the comfort of your chair.

1. Journey Through the Desert

- Inspiration: Imagine the vast, open skies and the warm, golden sands of the desert.

- Poses: Begin with Sun Salutations modified for chair yoga to welcome the warmth of the sun. Transition to cactus arms to mimic the resilient desert flora, opening your chest and embracing the vastness. A seated camel pose invites you to explore the sensation of heat and endurance, stretching your front body and lifting your heart towards the sky.

2. Explore the Rainforest

- Inspiration: Envision the lush, dense foliage and the vibrant life within a tropical rainforest.

- Poses: Incorporate twisting poses to represent the winding vines and the dynamic life forms. Use arm raises and overhead stretches to emulate the towering trees reaching for sunlight. Bird poses adapted for chair yoga can reflect the diverse avian life, focusing on balance and the lightness of being.

3. Sojourn in the Mountains

- Inspiration: Picture the majestic peaks and serene landscapes of mountain ranges.

- Poses: Mountain pose in a chair sets the foundation, embodying solidity and strength. Move into a seated version of the Warrior poses, visualizing the ascent up steep trails and the exhilaration of reaching the summit. Incorporate arm extensions and side bends to emulate the expansive views and the freedom of the high altitudes.

4. Sail Across the Seas

- Inspiration: Imagine the rhythmic waves and the boundless horizons of the ocean.

- Poses: Begin with seated forward and back bends to mimic the ebb and flow of the tides. Twisting poses can represent the navigation through changing currents. Finish with a relaxation pose, allowing the gentle motion to lull you into a state of peacefulness, as if floating on calm waters.

5. Wander Through a Meadow

- Inspiration: Visualize a peaceful meadow, dotted with wildflowers and bathed in sunlight.

- Poses: Flower poses and gentle seated stretches can symbolize the blooming flowers and the soft grass. Incorporate gentle side bends and arm flows to mimic the breeze swaying through the meadow. End with a visualization meditation, imagining the colors, scents, and sounds of this tranquil setting.

By incorporating these imaginative sequences into your chair yoga practice, you create an opportunity for mental travel and exploration that transcends physical limitations. Each journey offers a unique way to connect with different elements of nature and the world, enhancing your practice with creativity, relaxation, and joy. This approach not only benefits the body but also nourishes the soul, reminding us of the boundless adventures that await in the realms of our imagination.

Wellness Through Movement

Chair yoga stands as a beacon of accessibility and gentleness in the vast sea of wellness practices, offering a bridge to improved mental and physical health for individuals of all ages and abilities. This form of yoga, tailored to be performed while seated or using a chair for support, demystifies the notion that one must be highly flexible, strong, or even standing to reap the benefits of yoga. Let's delve into the myriad ways chair yoga nurtures both body and mind, alongside practical tips to weave this practice into the tapestry of your daily wellness routine.

Supporting Physical Health

Chair yoga makes the extensive benefits of traditional yoga accessible, especially for those who might find standing poses challenging. Here's how it supports physical health:

- Enhanced Flexibility: Regular practice gently stretches and elongates the muscles, which can reduce stiffness and increase the range of motion in joints. Movements designed for the arms, legs, and spine help maintain or improve flexibility, crucial for daily activities and overall mobility.

- Improved Strength: Through various seated or standing poses that use the chair for support, individuals engage multiple muscle groups. This engagement, even in a gentle form, helps build and maintain muscle strength, contributing to better posture, balance, and bodily functions.

- Increased Balance: Balance is a critical component of physical health, particularly as we age. Chair yoga incorporates poses that enhance core strength and stability, reducing the risk of falls and improving the ability to perform daily tasks.

- Promotion of Joint Health: Gentle movements and stretches can lubricate joints, increase blood circulation, and help manage or alleviate pain associated with conditions like arthritis.

Nurturing Mental Health

The mental health benefits of chair yoga are profound and multifaceted, touching on aspects of stress reduction, mindfulness, and emotional well-being:

- Stress Reduction: Through focused breathing exercises and mindful movement, chair yoga promotes relaxation and stress relief. The practice encourages the activation of the parasympathetic nervous system, often referred to as the "rest and digest" system, which can help lower stress levels and induce a state of calm.

- Improved Focus and Clarity: The meditative aspects of chair yoga, combined with breathing exercises, can enhance mental clarity and concentration. This practice encourages a mindfulness that can reduce cognitive decline and boost cognitive functions.

- Emotional Balance: Engaging in chair yoga can lead to an increase in serotonin levels, often dubbed the "happiness hormone," which plays a part in mood regulation. The practice also teaches coping mechanisms for anxiety and depression, promoting emotional resilience.

Incorporating Chair Yoga into Your Wellness Routine

- Start Small: Begin with a short daily practice, perhaps 10-15 minutes, and gradually increase as you become more comfortable. Consistency is key to experiencing the benefits.

- Make It a Habit: Incorporate chair yoga into your daily routine at a specific time that works for you, making it as habitual as having your morning coffee or reading before bed.

- Use Resources: Take advantage of books, online videos, and community classes designed for chair yoga. These resources can provide guidance, variety, and support as you explore different poses and sequences.

- Listen to Your Body: Chair yoga is about meeting your body where it is. Adapt poses as needed, and always practice with mindfulness to avoid discomfort or injury.

- Combine with Other Wellness Practices: Integrate chair yoga with other aspects of wellness, such as healthy eating, meditation, or outdoor walks, to create a holistic approach to health and well-being.

Chair yoga exemplifies how movement, even when adapted to be gentle and accessible, can be a powerful catalyst for health and happiness. By embracing this practice, individuals can embark on a journey of wellness that nourishes the body, calms the mind, and uplifts the spirit.

Starting a Chair Yoga Group

Embarking on the journey of chair yoga can be a deeply personal experience, yet sharing this path with others can magnify its benefits, creating a sense of community and collective growth. Starting a chair yoga group, whether locally in your community or online, offers a wonderful opportunity to connect with peers, share experiences, and support each other in the pursuit of wellness. Forming such a group might seem daunting at first, but with a few thoughtful steps, you can create a space that welcomes all levels of experience and fosters a shared journey of health and mindfulness.

The first step in creating a chair yoga group is to identify the potential members of your community who might be interested. This could include friends, family members, or neighbors, particularly those who might benefit from a gentle form of exercise due to mobility issues, health concerns, or simply a desire for a more accessible approach to yoga. Reaching out through community centers, local libraries, or social media platforms can help widen your circle and invite individuals who share your interest in chair yoga.

Once you've gathered a group of interested individuals, the next step is to decide on the format and setting of your meetings. For a local group, consider spaces that are accessible and comfortable for all participants, such as community centers, church halls, or even a spacious living room. It's important to ensure that the chosen space is conducive to practicing yoga, with enough room for each participant to move freely in their chair without obstruction. If you're leaning towards forming an online group, platforms like Zoom or Skype can offer a convenient way to connect from the comfort of your own homes, allowing for flexibility in scheduling and participation from a wider geographical area.

Establishing a regular schedule is crucial for maintaining the momentum and commitment of the group. Whether meeting once a week or more frequently, consistency helps build a routine that members can look forward to. It also provides structure to the group's activities, ensuring that each session builds upon the last and offers a progressive journey through the practices of chair yoga.

Leading a chair yoga group does not require you to be an expert or certified yoga instructor, though having someone with experience in guiding yoga practices can be beneficial. The focus should be on creating a supportive environment where everyone feels comfortable to participate at their own pace. Utilizing resources such as instructional videos, books, or even inviting guest instructors for special sessions can enhance the group's experience and provide a variety of perspectives on chair yoga practices.

As the group evolves, encourage feedback and suggestions from members to tailor the sessions to the group's needs and interests. Creating a sense of ownership and shared responsibility can foster a strong community bond, making the chair yoga group not just about practicing yoga, but about building relationships and supporting each other's wellness journeys.

In forming a chair yoga group, you're not just facilitating a space for physical activity, but also creating a community that values health, mindfulness, and mutual support. It's a journey that goes beyond the individual, embracing the collective power of shared experiences and the transformative impact of chair yoga on both body and mind.

Sharing the Joy

Sharing the joy of yoga with friends and family can transform it from a solitary practice into a rich, communal experience that benefits everyone involved. The key to encouraging those around you to join in lies in demonstrating the positive impact it has had on your own life, without pushing or insisting too strongly. Often, the best encouragement comes from simply embodying the peace, strength, and vitality that yoga brings into your life. When friends and family see the positive changes in you, they may become curious and more willing to give it a try themselves.

Start by sharing your own yoga journey in a way that highlights the benefits you've experienced, be it improved flexibility, reduced stress, better sleep, or simply a greater sense of calm and well-being. Personal stories and experiences can be powerful motivators, especially when they come from a place of genuine enthusiasm and love.

Another effective approach is to invite them to join you in a non-intimidating, welcoming environment. This could be a beginner's class at a local studio, a gentle chair yoga session at home, or even a virtual class where they can participate from the comfort of their own space. Make it clear that yoga is a practice where everyone starts somewhere, and there's no expectation to be perfect or to perform complex poses right away. The focus is on the journey, not the destination.

You might also consider making it a social activity, where the practice of yoga is followed by something enjoyable, like sharing a meal or going for a walk together. This creates a positive association with the practice and turns it into an opportunity for quality time together, rather than just another fitness routine.

It's also helpful to address any misconceptions they may have about yoga. Many people hesitate to try yoga because they believe they're not flexible enough, too old, or that yoga is too spiritual for their taste. By explaining the variety of yoga styles and the adaptability of practices like chair yoga, you can help dispel these myths and show that yoga truly is for everyone.

Finally, practice patience and understanding. Everyone's journey to yoga is unique, and it may take time for your loved ones to find their path to the mat. The most important thing is to keep the invitation open, offering support and information whenever they show interest. Remember, the goal is to share something you love, not to convince them to adopt a practice they're not ready for.

By sharing the joys and benefits of yoga in a loving, open-hearted manner, you create the opportunity for your friends and family to explore a practice that enhances life in countless ways. Whether they join you for one session or become lifelong yoga enthusiasts, the act of sharing something so meaningful can deepen your relationships and bring a new dimension of connection and joy to your lives.

Staying Motivated

Maintaining motivation for a consistent yoga practice can sometimes be challenging, but with the right strategies, yoga can become an enjoyable and lasting part of your lifestyle. The journey begins with setting realistic expectations and goals for your practice. Understanding that yoga is more than just physical exercise—it's a path to physical, mental, and emotional well-being—can help in appreciating each session, regardless of its intensity or duration. This holistic view encourages a deeper commitment, making it easier to integrate yoga into your daily life.

One effective way to stay motivated is to vary your practice. Exploring different styles of yoga, incorporating various poses, or even changing the time and place of your practice can keep things interesting. This variety not only challenges your body in new ways but also keeps your mind engaged. You might find that certain styles resonate more with you on particular days, depending on your mood, energy levels, and physical needs. Listening to your body and allowing your practice to be flexible can lead to a more satisfying and sustainable yoga journey.

Creating a dedicated space for your practice can also enhance your motivation. This doesn't necessarily mean you need a large room or special equipment; even a small, quiet corner where you can roll out your mat can become a sanctuary for your practice. This dedicated space can serve as a visual reminder and an invitation to practice, making it easier to step onto the mat even when motivation is low.

Incorporating yoga into your routine is another strategy for maintaining motivation. Just as you schedule time for meals, work, and social activities, scheduling specific times for yoga can help in making it a non-negotiable part of your day. Over time, this consistency builds a habit, making it feel as natural as brushing your teeth or having your morning coffee.

Connecting with the yoga community, whether online or in person, can offer additional motivation. Sharing your experiences, challenges, and successes with others who are on a similar path can provide encouragement, inspiration, and a sense of belonging. This community connection can be particularly motivating on days when your personal commitment might waver.

Finally, focusing on the benefits you're experiencing from your practice can be a powerful motivator. Whether it's improved flexibility, reduced stress, better sleep, or a greater sense of inner peace, acknowledging these positive changes can reinforce your commitment to your practice. Keeping a journal where you reflect on these benefits can serve as a helpful reminder of why you started yoga and why it's worth continuing.

By integrating these strategies into your approach to yoga, you can transform it from a sporadic activity into a cherished part of your lifestyle. The key is to remain patient and compassionate with yourself, allowing your practice to evolve naturally over time. With this mindset, yoga can become a source of joy, growth, and well-being that you look forward to every day.

Learning More

For those interested in deepening their chair yoga practice, several resources can enrich your journey, offering insights from foundational techniques to advanced practices. Here are some recommended books, each providing a unique perspective on yoga:

- "The Complete Guide to Yin Yoga" by Bernie Clark dives into the slow-paced style of Yin Yoga, where poses are held for longer periods, focusing on deep stretching and mindfulness. This book is particularly beneficial for understanding the meditative and restorative aspects of yoga, making it suitable for practitioners looking to deepen their practice beyond the physical postures.

- "Restorative Yoga for Life" by Gail Grossman explores the gentle, healing side of yoga, emphasizing the use of props to support the body in various poses fully. This approach allows for deep relaxation and rejuvenation, making it an excellent resource for those seeking to incorporate a calming, therapeutic element into their routine.

- "Ashtanga Yoga: The Practice Manual" by David Swenson provides a comprehensive look at the Ashtanga Yoga system, known for its dynamic and physically demanding sequence of poses. This manual is a valuable resource for practitioners interested in exploring a more vigorous style of yoga, with detailed instructions and modifications for each pose.

- "The Heart of Yoga" by T.K.V. Desikachar delves into the philosophy and spiritual aspects of yoga, offering insights into how to integrate yoga principles into daily life. The book includes a translation of Patanjali's Yoga Sutras, providing a foundational understanding of yoga's ethical and philosophical core.

- "Living Your Yoga" by Judith Lasater discusses how to apply yoga's lessons beyond the mat, touching on themes like relaxation, empathy, and worship. Lasater's approach encourages readers to bring yoga principles into every aspect of their lives, promoting a holistic practice that nurtures body, mind, and spirit.

- "Wheels of Life" by Anodea Judith offers an in-depth exploration of the chakra system, linking yoga practice with the body's energetic centers. This book is ideal for those interested in the intersection of yoga and energy work, providing practical guidance for balancing and activating the chakras through yoga.

- "The Extended Chair for Yoga: A Comprehensive Guide to Iyengar Yoga Practice with a Chair" by Eyal Shifroni specifically targets those interested in chair yoga, offering an extensive array of adaptations for traditional poses using a chair. This book is particularly useful for yoga practitioners and teachers looking to make yoga accessible to everyone, regardless of mobility or experience level.

Each of these books offers a unique perspective on yoga, catering to different interests and aspects of the practice. Whether you're drawn to the physical, philosophical, or therapeutic elements of yoga, these resources can guide you toward a deeper, more fulfilling practice.

Conclusion

Embarking on the path of chair yoga is much more than a journey into a physical practice; it's an exploration into the depths of self-discovery and a celebration of joy that transcends the boundaries of physical health. This gentle form of yoga invites us to meet ourselves exactly where we are, offering a unique opportunity to engage with our bodies and minds in a compassionate and nurturing way. Chair yoga is not merely about achieving better flexibility or strength, though these are certainly valuable benefits. More profoundly, it's about uncovering layers of ourselves, learning to listen to our bodies with kindness, and discovering what it means to move in harmony with our own rhythms.

As we fold into a seated forward bend or stretch our arms in a seated mountain pose, we're not just going through the motions; we're engaging in a dialogue with the deepest parts of ourselves. This practice becomes a mirror, reflecting back to us our resilience, our challenges, and our capacity for growth and change. It teaches us patience and perseverance, as we learn to embrace our limitations and celebrate our progress, no matter how small it might seem.

Moreover, chair yoga offers a pathway to joy, an often overlooked aspect of wellness. In the simplicity of breath and movement, there's a profound capacity for joy to emerge. As we breathe deeply, stretching into each pose with intention, we might find moments of pure presence, where the mind quiets and the heart opens. These moments, though fleeting, remind us of the joy inherent in simply being alive, in being able to move and breathe with awareness.

The personal gains from chair yoga extend far beyond physical health, touching the essence of who we are. This practice invites us into a deeper relationship with ourselves, one that honors our wholeness and our humanity. It's a journey that asks us to show up for ourselves, to nurture our well-being with each breath and each pose. In doing so, we discover that chair yoga is not just a practice for the body, but a celebration of life itself, offering us tools to live more fully, with greater joy and a deeper sense of connection to ourselves.

Thus, I encourage you to view chair yoga not just as an exercise regimen, but as a journey of self-discovery and joy. Let it be a practice that enriches your life, offering personal gains that resonate far beyond physical health, illuminating the path to a more joyful, vibrant, and connected way of living.

Made in the USA
Coppell, TX
11 May 2025

49203023R10059